Reverse PCOS

Polycystic Ovarian Syndrome Treatment Diet Plans to Loose Weight and Boost Fertility

Maya Arlo

TABLE OF CONTENTS

Chapter 7: Monitoring Progress and Making Adjustments to the Diet Plan as Needed for Optimal PCOS Management

Chapter 1

Understanding Polycystic Ovarian Syndrome (PCOS)

Polycystic Ovarian Syndrome (PCOS) is a common hormonal disorder that affects many women of reproductive age. It is estimated that up to 10% of women worldwide have PCOS, making it one of the most common endocrine disorders in women. PCOS is characterized by a range of symptoms that can impact a woman's health and wellbeing, including irregular periods, excessive hair growth, acne, and weight gain. It is also a leading cause of infertility in women.

In this chapter, we will explore the causes and symptoms of PCOS, as well as the diagnostic criteria used to identify the condition. We will also look at the impact that PCOS can have on a woman's overall health, including the increased risk of other health conditions such as diabetes and cardiovascular disease.

What is Polycystic Ovarian Syndrome (PCOS)?

Polycystic Ovarian Syndrome (PCOS) is a hormonal disorder that affects women of reproductive age. It is characterized by the presence of multiple cysts on the ovaries, which can disrupt the normal functioning of the ovaries and result in a range of symptoms. The exact cause of PCOS is not yet fully understood, but it is believed to be a combination of genetic and environmental factors.

Symptoms of PCOS

The symptoms of PCOS can vary widely between individuals, but the most common symptoms include:

Irregular periods: Women with PCOS may experience irregular or absent periods, which can make it difficult to predict ovulation and make it harder to conceive.

Excessive hair growth: PCOS can cause excessive hair growth in areas such as the face, chest, and back. This is due to the increased production of androgens, which are male hormones that are also present in women.

Acne: PCOS can cause acne, especially on the face, chest, and back.

Weight gain: Women with PCOS are more likely to gain weight and find it difficult to lose weight. This is due to the insulin resistance that is often associated with PCOS.

Infertility: PCOS is a leading cause of infertility in women. The hormonal imbalances associated with PCOS can disrupt ovulation and make it difficult to conceive.

Diagnosis of PCOS

There is no single test that can diagnose PCOS. Instead, doctors will look for a combination of symptoms and perform certain tests to rule out other conditions. The diagnostic criteria for PCOS are:

Irregular periods: Women with PCOS may have fewer than eight menstrual cycles per year, or they may have periods that are irregular in length.

Excessive androgen levels: Women with PCOS often have higher levels of androgens than normal. This can be detected through a blood test.

Ovarian cysts: Women with PCOS may have multiple cysts on their ovaries, which can be detected through an ultrasound.

Impact of PCOS on Overall Health

PCOS can have a significant impact on a woman's overall health and wellbeing. Women with PCOS are at an increased risk of developing a range of health conditions, including:

Diabetes: Women with PCOS are more likely to develop type 2 diabetes, due to the insulin resistance that is often associated with PCOS.

Cardiovascular disease: PCOS is associated with an increased risk of cardiovascular disease, including high blood pressure and high cholesterol.

Endometrial cancer: Women with PCOS may be at an increased risk of developing endometrial cancer, due to the disruption of ovulation and the increased production of estrogen.

Chapter 2

Understanding the Role of Diet in Managing PCOS Symptoms

Polycystic Ovarian Syndrome (PCOS) is a hormonal disorder that can cause a range of symptoms, including weight gain, irregular periods, and infertility. While there is no cure for PCOS, there are several lifestyle changes that can help manage symptoms, including diet modifications. In this chapter, we will explore the role of diet in managing PCOS symptoms, including the types of foods that can help alleviate symptoms and the foods that should be avoided.

The Link Between Diet and PCOS

Diet plays a crucial role in managing PCOS symptoms. Studies have shown that women with PCOS are more likely to have insulin resistance, which can lead to high blood sugar levels and weight gain. Insulin resistance occurs when the body's cells become less responsive to insulin, a hormone that regulates blood sugar levels. This can lead to an increase in the production of androgens, which can cause symptoms such as acne, excessive hair growth, and irregular periods.

Eating a healthy, balanced diet can help manage insulin resistance and improve symptoms associated with PCOS. The right foods can also help regulate hormone levels and reduce inflammation in the body, which can help alleviate symptoms such as acne and excessive hair growth.

Foods to Include in a PCOS Diet

High-fiber foods: Fiber helps regulate blood sugar levels and can improve insulin sensitivity. Good sources of fiber include whole grains, fruits, and vegetables.

Lean protein: Protein can help you feel full and satisfied, which can help with weight management. Good sources of lean protein include chicken, fish, and tofu.

Healthy fats: Fats are an important part of a balanced diet and can help regulate hormone levels. Good sources of healthy fats include nuts, seeds, avocado, and olive oil.

Low-glycemic index foods: Foods with a low glycemic index (GI) are digested more slowly, which can help regulate blood sugar levels. Good sources of low-GI foods include whole grains, legumes, and non-starchy vegetables.

Foods to Avoid in a PCOS Diet

Sugary foods and drinks: Sugary foods and drinks can cause blood sugar levels to spike, which can worsen insulin resistance. This includes soda, candy, and desserts.

Processed foods: Processed foods are often high in added sugars and unhealthy fats, which can contribute to weight gain and inflammation in the body.

High-glycemic index foods: Foods with a high GI can cause blood sugar levels to spike, which can worsen insulin resistance. This includes white bread, white rice, and pasta.

Dairy products: Some studies have shown that dairy products may worsen symptoms of PCOS, such as acne and irregular periods.

Implementing a PCOS Diet

When implementing a PCOS diet, it is important to focus on whole, nutrient-dense foods and to limit processed and sugary foods. Eating regular meals and snacks throughout the day can also help regulate blood sugar levels and improve insulin sensitivity.

In addition to making dietary changes, regular exercise can also help manage PCOS symptoms. Exercise can help improve insulin sensitivity and regulate hormone levels, which can lead to a reduction in symptoms such as weight gain and acne.

Diet plays a crucial role in managing PCOS symptoms. Eating a balanced diet that is rich in fiber, lean protein, and healthy fats can help regulate blood sugar levels and improve insulin sensitivity.

Avoiding sugary and processed foods, as well as high-GI foods and dairy products, can also help manage PCOS symptoms. By making dietary changes and incorporating regular exercise into your routine, you can help alleviate symptoms and improve your overall health and wellbeing.

Chapter 3

Creating a Personalized Diet Plan for PCOS Patients to Promote Weight Loss and Improve Fertility

Polycystic Ovarian Syndrome (PCOS) is a hormonal disorder that can cause a range of symptoms, including weight gain, irregular periods, and infertility.

While there is no cure for PCOS, a personalized diet plan can help manage symptoms and improve fertility. In this chapter, we will explore how to create a personalized diet plan for PCOS patients to promote weight loss and improve fertility.

Assessing Your Nutritional Needs

The first step in creating a personalized diet plan for PCOS patients is to assess your nutritional needs. This involves evaluating your current diet and identifying areas for improvement. You may also want to consider working with a registered dietitian who has experience working with PCOS patients.

When assessing your nutritional needs, it is important to consider your age, height, weight, and activity level. You should also take into account any medical conditions or medications that may affect your nutritional needs. For example, some medications used to treat PCOS can increase the risk of vitamin B12 deficiency.

Designing Your PCOS Diet Plan

Once you have assessed your nutritional needs, you can begin to design your PCOS diet plan. A well-designed PCOS diet plan should include foods that promote weight loss and improve fertility.

Promoting weight loss: Weight loss is an important aspect of managing PCOS symptoms. Losing even a small amount of weight can improve insulin sensitivity and regulate hormone levels. To promote weight loss, your diet should include foods that are low in calories but high in fiber and protein. This includes fruits, vegetables, lean proteins, and whole grains.

Improving fertility: Many women with PCOS struggle with fertility issues. To improve fertility, your diet should include foods that support reproductive health.

This includes foods that are rich in antioxidants, such as berries, leafy greens, and nuts. You should also make sure to include foods that are rich in iron, such as lean red meat and leafy greens, as iron deficiency can contribute to infertility.

Regulating blood sugar levels: As previously mentioned, many women with PCOS have insulin resistance, which can lead to high blood sugar levels and weight gain. To regulate blood sugar levels, your diet should include foods that are low in sugar and high in fiber. This includes non-starchy vegetables, whole grains, and legumes.

Incorporating healthy fats: Healthy fats are an important part of a balanced diet and can help regulate hormone levels. This includes foods such as nuts, seeds, avocado, and olive oil.

Meal Planning and Preparation

Once you have designed your PCOS diet plan, it is important to create a meal plan and prepare meals ahead of time. This can help you stay on track and avoid making unhealthy food choices when you are pressed for time.

When meal planning, it is important to make sure that your meals are balanced and include a variety of nutrient-dense foods. You should also make sure to include snacks throughout the day to help regulate blood sugar levels and prevent overeating.

Preparing meals ahead of time can also help you save time and reduce stress. This can involve prepping ingredients ahead of time, cooking meals in batches, and storing leftovers for future meals.

A personalized diet plan can help manage symptoms and improve fertility for PCOS patients. When designing your PCOS diet plan, it is important to consider your nutritional needs and incorporate foods that promote weight loss, improve fertility, regulate blood sugar levels, and incorporate healthy fats. Meal planning and preparation can also help you stay on track and make healthy food choices throughout the week. By working with a registered dietitian and implementing a personalized diet plan, you can help manage PCOS symptoms and improve your overall health and wellbeing

Chapter 4

Incorporating Exercise and Physical Activity into a PCOS Treatment Plan

Polycystic Ovarian Syndrome (PCOS) is a hormonal disorder that can cause a range of symptoms, including weight gain, irregular periods, and infertility. While there is no cure for PCOS, incorporating exercise and physical activity into a treatment plan can help manage symptoms and improve overall health. In this chapter, we will explore the benefits of exercise for PCOS patients and how to incorporate it into a treatment plan.

Benefits of Exercise for PCOS Patients

Exercise has numerous benefits for PCOS patients, including:

Weight loss: Exercise can help promote weight loss, which is an important aspect of managing PCOS symptoms. Losing even a small amount of weight can improve insulin sensitivity and regulate hormone levels.

Regulation of blood sugar levels: Exercise can help regulate blood sugar levels by increasing insulin sensitivity.

Improved fertility: Exercise can help improve fertility by promoting weight loss and regulating hormone levels.

Reduction in inflammation: PCOS is associated with chronic inflammation, which can lead to a range of health issues. Exercise can help reduce inflammation and improve overall health.

Improved mental health: Exercise is known to improve mood and reduce symptoms of anxiety and depression.

Designing an Exercise Program for PCOS Patients

When designing an exercise program for PCOS patients, it is important to consider their fitness level and any medical conditions or injuries that may affect their ability to exercise.

Cardiovascular exercise: Cardiovascular exercise, such as walking, jogging, cycling, or swimming, is an effective way to promote weight loss and improve cardiovascular health. Aim for at least 30 minutes of moderate-intensity exercise most days of the week.

Strength training: Strength training is an important component of an exercise program for PCOS patients. It can help build muscle mass, which can increase metabolism and promote weight loss. Aim for 2-3 strength training sessions per week.

High-intensity interval training (HIIT): HIIT is a form of exercise that involves short bursts of high-intensity exercise followed by periods of rest. This type of exercise has been shown to be effective for promoting weight loss and improving insulin sensitivity.

Yoga and Pilates: Yoga and Pilates are low-impact exercises that can help improve flexibility, reduce stress, and improve overall health.

Tips for Incorporating Exercise into a PCOS Treatment Plan

Incorporating exercise into a PCOS treatment plan can be challenging, but there are a few tips that can help make it easier:

Start slowly: If you are new to exercise, start slowly and gradually increase the intensity and duration of your workouts.

Find activities you enjoy: Exercise should be enjoyable and sustainable. Try different types of exercise until you find something you enjoy.

Make it a habit: Set a regular schedule for exercise and make it a habit. This can help make exercise a regular part of your routine.

Get support: Enlist the support of friends, family, or a personal trainer to help you stay motivated and accountable.

Incorporating exercise and physical activity into a PCOS treatment plan can help manage symptoms and improve overall health. Exercise can promote weight loss, regulate blood sugar levels, improve fertility, reduce inflammation, and improve mental health. By designing an exercise program that is tailored to your fitness level and interests, and by following the tips outlined in this chapter, you can make exercise a regular part of your PCOS treatment plan and improve your overall health and wellbeing.

Chapter 5

The Role of Supplements and Herbal Remedies in Managing PCOS Symptoms

Polycystic Ovarian Syndrome (PCOS) is a hormonal disorder that affects many women worldwide. While there is no cure for PCOS, lifestyle modifications such as diet and exercise, and medication can help manage symptoms. Another approach that has gained popularity in recent years is the use of supplements and herbal remedies. In this chapter, we will explore the role of supplements and herbal remedies in managing PCOS symptoms.

Understanding Supplements and Herbal Remedies

Supplements and herbal remedies are products that are taken orally and are meant to supplement the diet or treat a specific health condition. They can come in various forms, including capsules, tablets, powders, teas, and tinctures. The ingredients in these products can range from vitamins and minerals to herbs and botanicals.

While supplements and herbal remedies can have health benefits, it is important to remember that they are not regulated by the Food and Drug Administration (FDA) in the same way as prescription medications. This means that the safety and effectiveness of these products are not always guaranteed. Before starting any supplement or herbal remedy, it is important to consult with a healthcare provider and ensure it is safe and appropriate for you.

Supplements for PCOS

Several supplements have been studied for their potential benefits in managing PCOS symptoms. Here are some of the most commonly used supplements for PCOS:

Inositol: Inositol is a type of sugar that has been shown to improve insulin resistance and regulate hormone levels in women with PCOS. It is available in supplement form and is often used to promote ovulation and improve fertility.

Omega-3 fatty acids: Omega-3 fatty acids are essential fatty acids found in fish, nuts, and seeds. They have been shown to reduce inflammation, regulate blood sugar levels, and improve cardiovascular health in women with PCOS.

Vitamin D: Vitamin D is important for bone health and immune function. Women with PCOS are at a higher risk for vitamin D deficiency, which can worsen insulin resistance and increase the risk of cardiovascular disease. Supplementing with vitamin D may help improve these symptoms.

Chromium: Chromium is a mineral that has been shown to improve insulin sensitivity and regulate blood sugar levels in women with PCOS.

N-acetylcysteine (NAC): NAC is an antioxidant that has been shown to improve insulin resistance and reduce inflammation in women with PCOS.

Herbal Remedies for PCOS

Herbal remedies have been used for centuries to treat a variety of health conditions. While scientific research on herbal remedies for PCOS is limited, some herbs have been shown to have potential benefits in managing symptoms. Here are some of the most commonly used herbal remedies for PCOS:

Cinnamon: Cinnamon is a spice that has been shown to improve insulin sensitivity and regulate blood sugar levels in women with PCOS.

Licorice: Licorice is a root that has been shown to improve ovulation and reduce inflammation in women with PCOS.

Spearmint: Spearmint is a type of mint that has been shown to reduce androgen levels in women with PCOS.

Saw palmetto: Saw palmetto is a berry that has been shown to reduce androgen levels in women with PCOS.

Chasteberry: Chasteberry is a fruit that has been shown to improve menstrual cycle regularity and reduce symptoms of PMS in women with PCOS.

Supplements and herbal remedies can be a helpful addition to a PCOS treatment plan, but it is important to remember that they are not a substitute for medical treatment or lifestyle modifications.

Chapter

6

Strategies for Overcoming Common Challenges in Adhering to a PCOS Treatment Diet Plan

Polycystic Ovarian Syndrome (PCOS) is a hormonal disorder that affects many women worldwide. While lifestyle modifications, including a healthy diet, are crucial for managing PCOS symptoms, adhering to a diet plan can be challenging. In this chapter, we will explore strategies for overcoming common challenges in adhering to a PCOS treatment diet plan.

Challenge 1: Cravings and Emotional Eating

One of the most significant challenges in adhering to a PCOS treatment diet plan is cravings and emotional eating. Many women with PCOS struggle with cravings for sugar, carbs, and high-fat foods, which can be hard to resist. Additionally, stress, anxiety, and other emotions can lead to emotional eating, which can derail a diet plan.

Solution: The key to overcoming cravings and emotional eating is to identify triggers and develop coping mechanisms. Keeping a food diary and noting when cravings occur can help identify triggers. Additionally, finding healthy ways to cope with emotions, such as exercise, meditation, or talking to a friend, can help avoid emotional eating.

Challenge 2: Social Events and Dining Out

Social events and dining out can be challenging when following a PCOS treatment diet plan. Many social events revolve around food, and it can be challenging to find healthy options at restaurants.

Solution: When dining out, it is essential to plan ahead. Researching menus in advance, choosing restaurants that offer healthy options, and requesting modifications can help stay on track with a diet plan. Additionally, bringing healthy snacks to social events and focusing on the social aspect of the event rather than the food can help stay on track.

Challenge 3: Time and Convenience

Many women with PCOS struggle with time and convenience when it comes to meal planning and preparation. Busy schedules can make it challenging to find time to prepare healthy meals, leading to reliance on fast food and processed snacks.

Solution: Meal planning and preparation can help overcome the challenge of time and convenience. Scheduling time to plan meals and grocery shop can ensure that healthy ingredients are always on hand. Additionally, preparing meals in advance, such as on weekends, can save time during busy weekdays.

Challenge 4: Lack of Support

Lack of support from friends and family can make it challenging to adhere to a PCOS treatment diet plan. Negative comments, pressure to eat unhealthy foods, and lack of understanding can make it challenging to stay motivated.

Solution: Finding support is crucial for success in adhering to a PCOS treatment diet plan. Seeking support from a healthcare provider, joining a support group, or enlisting the help of friends and family can provide motivation and accountability.

Challenge 5: Boredom and Lack of Variety

Eating the same foods repeatedly and lack of variety can make a PCOS treatment diet plan boring and unappealing.

Solution: Adding variety to meals can help overcome the challenge of boredom and lack of variety. Trying new recipes, experimenting with different cuisines, and incorporating a variety of healthy ingredients can help keep meals interesting and appealing.

Adhering to a PCOS treatment diet plan can be challenging, but with the right strategies, it is possible to overcome common challenges. Identifying triggers, planning ahead, finding support, adding variety, and developing coping mechanisms can all help stay on track with a diet plan. By making lifestyle modifications and adhering to a healthy diet, women with PCOS can effectively manage symptoms and improve overall health.

Chapter 7

Monitoring Progress and Making Adjustments to the Diet Plan as Needed for Optimal PCOS Management

Polycystic Ovarian Syndrome (PCOS) is a complex hormonal disorder that requires a comprehensive management plan. In addition to making lifestyle modifications, including diet and exercise, it is important to regularly monitor progress and make adjustments as needed to ensure optimal PCOS management. In this chapter, we will explore the importance of monitoring progress and making adjustments to the diet plan for PCOS management.

Why is Monitoring Progress Important for PCOS Management?

Monitoring progress is essential for PCOS management because it allows for early detection of changes in symptoms and the effectiveness of treatment. Regular monitoring can help identify patterns and trends in symptoms, such as changes in menstrual cycles, weight, and acne, which can guide adjustments to the treatment plan. Additionally, tracking progress can provide motivation and accountability for adhering to a healthy diet and lifestyle.

How to Monitor Progress for PCOS Management?

There are several ways to monitor progress for PCOS management, including:

Keeping a Food Diary: Keeping a food diary can help track food intake, identify trigger foods, and monitor adherence to a healthy diet plan.

Tracking Body Weight: Monitoring body weight can help track progress in weight loss or weight gain, which is important for managing PCOS symptoms.

Measuring Body Composition: Measuring body composition, including body fat percentage and muscle mass, can provide a more accurate assessment of progress than simply tracking body weight.

Monitoring Menstrual Cycles: Monitoring menstrual cycles can help identify changes in cycle length and regularity, which are important indicators of hormonal balance.

Checking Hormone Levels: Checking hormone levels, including testosterone, estrogen, and insulin, can provide insight into the effectiveness of treatment and guide adjustments to the treatment plan.

Making Adjustments to the Diet Plan for Optimal PCOS Management

Adjustments to the diet plan may be necessary for optimal PCOS management. Here are some common adjustments that may be needed:

Adjusting Macronutrient Ratios: The macronutrient ratios in a diet plan may need to be adjusted based on individual needs and preferences. For example, some women with PCOS may benefit from a higher protein or lower carbohydrate diet.

Adjusting Caloric Intake: Adjusting caloric intake may be necessary for weight loss or weight gain, which are important for managing PCOS symptoms.

Adding or Removing Specific Foods: Adding or removing specific foods may be necessary based on individual food intolerances, allergies, or preferences. For example, some women with PCOS may need to avoid dairy or gluten.

Incorporating Supplements: Incorporating supplements, such as omega-3 fatty acids or magnesium, may be beneficial for managing PCOS symptoms.

Adjusting Meal Timing: Adjusting meal timing, such as incorporating intermittent fasting, may be beneficial for improving insulin sensitivity and managing PCOS symptoms.

Conclusion

Monitoring progress and making adjustments to the diet plan are essential for optimal PCOS management. Regular monitoring can help identify changes in symptoms and guide adjustments to the treatment plan, while making adjustments to the diet plan can optimize the effectiveness of treatment. By working closely with a healthcare provider and regularly monitoring progress, women with PCOS can effectively manage symptoms and improve overall health.